The Revelation Diet

How to Miraculously Transform Your Body and Health Using Sound Biblical Methods!

By Patrick Doucette

The Revelation Diet

How to Miraculously Transform Your Body and Health Using Sound Biblical Methods!

By Patrick Doucette

Table of Contents

Introduction

You Can Do It! Yes, even if you have struggled with weight loss for as long as you can remember, this short simple book can show you how to achieve miraculous results with minimal effort! There is no other book like this available anywhere. The information has never been explained this way before – and now you have it in your grasp!

You may have given up on yourself; even if you believe you are destined to be fat for whatever reason your mind comes up with; this can all change with the information contained within these pages. The Revelation Diet will detail for you the simple principles that I followed to miraculously alter my body's ability to retain fat; in other words, following the principles of the

Revelation Diet caused the fat to melt off my body like the way ice cream melts in a sauna.

The Revelation Diet is not counting calories or a strict regimen that is impossible to follow. Instead it's a simple set of ideas that anyone can follow. Once you realize the power of these ideas, you'll want to share them with your friends and family and I encourage you to do just that.

You see, I also had my own mental mindset of why I was destined to be overweight. I believed that obesity was part of my family history and also that the stress of my job prevented me from being able to put any effort into weight control.

I can assure you that after reading this book, you will no longer have these mistaken beliefs that may be keeping you in the grip of an overweight prison.

Read this book! It will only take about an hour of your time and it can begin to transform your life. You may be tempted to toss this aside and tell yourself that it won't work; don't make that mistake! You owe it to yourself to check this out with your own eyes and your own mind.

I don't know how you found this book; perhaps a friend has shared it with you; perhaps it caught your eye on the internet somewhere - this may be your destined time; a golden opportunity to implement a solution that works for YOU!

Don't kick yourself, 3 months, 6 months or a year from now and wish you had read this book instead of just leaving it on a shelf! Read it today and then share it with a friend – you'll be glad you did!

Patrick

Doucette 2014

Chapter 1 - Oh Yes You Can!

Before we start, let me just say I know a new diet book is probably the last thing needed in the marketplace right now! How many diet books can you name just from memory alone? Probably quite a few! So why did I take the trouble to write this book for you? For a couple of reasons, first simply because I know it works; second because I have not seen or read anything like it and third and most importantly is because it will direct you towards your own path of self discovery.

Even though it has ideas that you can directly adopt and implement for your own health and benefit, I believe the best part of this message it that it will help many people to discover unique solutions that work best for themselves that simply cannot be gained by following a specific set of diet do's and don'ts.

A very short while ago, I was convinced that I was destined to be overweight. I knew that I was probably not going to be morbidly obese, for that I was certainly thankful. But because I saw other members of my immediate family and relatives that were overweight I felt that I too would be and indeed should be similar. This was not something I consciously acknowledged but I am certain it was an unconscious belief that was rooted deep in my mind. I had brothers and uncles with generous big pot bellies and aunts and cousins that were "big-boned." Now please understand I love my family and relatives dearly, and being overweight myself, I was never overly concerned about anything like an ideal weight. But deep down I was bit frustrated and embarrassed believing that "I was pre-destined to be overweight, and that's just the way it was."

All that changed for me in the spring of 2011. I had been praying for direction and asking God to provide me with the best solution for a healthy weight, when one day I began thinking of the Lord's Prayer. "Give us this day our daily bread..."

"Daily Bread." Hmm...I had never really thought about that prayer before but I starting thinking; what if we were only supposed to have one meal per day instead of three. I bet there are a lot of people in the world today that are lucky to get even one meal per day. We have been so accustomed to a breakfast, lunch and dinner routine that we take it for granted as a normal way to live.

I didn't think much of this at first and I tried to put it out of my mind. But the idea kept nagging at me again and again. "Give us this day our daily bread"...I decided I had to take some action. I bet you can guess what happened. I'm usually not that hungry in the morning so skipping breakfast was easy. I had a big lunch, probably too big and then tried to skip dinner. Of course I was climbing the walls all evening with hunger and could barely sleep. A disaster. This could not be what was meant in that familiar prayer I thought. I decided that 'daily bread' simply meant overall daily provision and decided to put it out of my mind.

But try as I might, I kept thinking that I had missed something. I also found a different message from Psalm 31 that encouraged me "...You will lead me and guide me." I felt these words were a real confirmation that I could depend on God for guidance in all things.

I felt a renewed encouragement that God was trying to tell me something. I returned to the idea of "Daily Bread" and decided to eat only one meal per day that had any bread or pasta. In other words if I had toast for breakfast, I would not eat any bread or pasta for the rest of the day. If I was planning to have pasta for dinner I would make sure that I would not eat any bread or pasta for breakfast or lunch. Success! This strategy only needed a minimal memory habit and I started to notice immediate improvement in my energy level. And here was the very start of what I like to call the 'Revelation Diet'.

You see, the Revelation Diet is not a specific set of food rules or an exact eating plan for everybody; rather the Revelation Diet is the process of discovering biblical principles of healthy eating that work for you as an individual. Even though I will give you a specific plan that I hope you will try in Chapter Seven – I believe that every individual is able to discover a unique that will work for them if they genuinely seek after it.

If 'the very hairs of our head are numbered', it only makes sense that God cares very much about our well being – and that includes whether we are overweight!

For some people, the idea of eating only one meal per day may work for them. For me, it did not and that's totally okay. It is obvious that we are all unique and that God wants us to be healthy. There is no benefit in being anorexic, suffering from bulimia or practicing excessive gluttony. Common sense tells us that a balanced diet is helpful and contributes to good health and happiness. Divine guidance is available to achieve this and that is what the Revelation Diet is all about! I want to share with you the unique revelations that have helped me and encourage you to find the unique revelations that will help you.

That is one of the most exciting things about depending on God for guidance is that we can expect to receive unique solutions! There are many examples of this in the bible that display this principle. Jesus did not heal everyone the same way. Some people were healed with a touch, others with a word and still others had specific instructions that were followed to enable the healing to occur. This is similar to what you will experience as you conquer the weight loss battle! Each unique solution is your own miracle and will bring you one step closer to a 'diet healing'!

Prayer for Chapter 1

"Dear God, please show me the best way to be healthy in body, mind and spirit. Please show me the dieting decisions that will work for me!" Amen.

Chapter 2 - The Problem With Me!

Whenever I tried to lose weight in the past, I would always experience a yo-yo effect or what I like to call 'the rubber-band effect'. That is where I would starve myself for a temporary period of time and then snap back all the weight I had lost in a single day. The point of failure inevitably involved a family gathering or a special occasion where I felt obligated to eat.

One year I ate only liquids during the entire forty days of Lent. I lost twenty pounds and gained it all back within 72 hours after starting solid food again. Another year I ate only unleavened bread for an entire week. My body had a violent reaction to that plan. I am a bit embarrassed to think of these failures now. They were not pleasant experiences but I was so anxious for weight loss that I was willing to try almost anything. My heart was sincere but I was following a bad strategy; that strategy was essentially a temporary change. I was reminded of the message from Mark 4:17 "...they have no firm root in themselves but are only temporary; then when affliction... arises because of the word, immediately they fall away..." I substituted 'food' for 'word' in that verse and saw my sorry state!

All my efforts had been only temporary! It was not until I found my 'daily bread' concept that I genuinely started to search for changes that could be permanent. I decided that I would only eat grain based foods; that is, breads, cereals or anything with wheat; only once per day. This was something that I knew I could incorporate as a permanent change. I decided to keep myself open to strategies that would work for me personally.

I decided that I would stop fooling myself and stop dieting. What a relief I felt! No more dieting, I said it out loud, "NO MORE DIETING!" It was a real burden lifted from off my shoulders – I no longer had to concern myself with temporary fixes. Instead I used this new found motivation to search out permanent changes. Using my 'daily bread principle' as a foundation I would start to build a way of eating and living that could not be shaken.

From now on I encourage you to give up dieting altogether! Yes, you heard that right; **stop trying to diet**. Dieting implies a temporary change. Trust me when I say that you do not need nor do you want a temporary change. You will find the key to victory in incremental permanent changes that by themselves may seem very small, but added together will become a powerful force towards a healthy and balanced lifestyle.

This subtle change in thinking can mean the difference between frustration and joyous victory! Take a moment to envision yourself as already healthy with an unwavering will. Any decisions you make from this day forward will not be under compulsion, they will not be temporary; no, instead the decisions you make will be because you are moving towards health and strength. From this day forward you will decide exactly how you want to implement change and you will only do things that you know will work for you.

Prayer for Chapter 2

"Dear God, please grant me the faith and strength to implement permanent changes in my eating habits that contribute towards healthy weight loss." Amen.

Chapter 3 - No Deadlines!

One of the first things that differentiated temporary change from permanent change was that temporary change always had deadlines! I was always trying to lose 5 pounds by this date or lose 10 pounds by that day. Temporary, temporary, temporary! From now on, I was only going to make changes that I knew should be and would be permanent.

My second breakthrough came in the summer of 2011. I was reading from Psalm 1 "He will be like a tree firmly planted by streams of **water**, which yields its fruit in its season and its leaf does not wither; and in whatever he does, he prospers." Water, the word jumped out at me. I had always heard about how important water is for proper health. Eight glasses per day and all that stuff, but I could never imagine myself drinking eight glasses of water per day; it made no sense to me. But suddenly I had another revelation about water. Water as a permanent change.

I knew that I drank soda too often; I knew that it was not good for me, even diet soda. Here I was spending money on diet soda when I could have healthy fresh water for free! I am still curious as to why I had become so passively addicted to commercial soft drinks without any thought. I made a conscious decision to start drinking water exclusively in place of soda. I now keep lemons on hand in the fridge and squeeze about a half ounce of lemon juice into a tall glass of water whenever I am thirsty.

I then extended this practice to fruit drinks. I realized that orange juice had a ton of sugar in it simply by reading the label; in fact it has as much or more than regular soda. Water became a permanent change. As I write this, I am still working on extending this to coffee. I used to drink three or four cups of coffee per day and I now only drink one cup in the morning. Soon, I will eliminate caffeine completely from my diet permanently. I know when it happens it will be a permanent change and I am in no rush and under no deadline but I am already excited by the positive results drinking more water has had on my health.

If I had breakfast with orange juice in the past, I would experience a real 'crash' in energy level by about ten or eleven in the morning. I am convinced it was from the large amount of sugar in the orange juice. I no longer have this energy drain but on the contrary I feel alert and vitalized throughout the day.

Trying to **add** more water to your diet will likely fail. At least it did for me. There was some type of forced compulsion that was similar to trying to stay on a specific diet. **Replacing** beverages with water, on the other hand, did not feel the same. There was no compulsion and almost no effort. I even saved some old juice containers and soda bottles and filled them with water and a splash of lemon juice. I'm not sure if this helped trick myself into making it a permanent change or not but it worked! I have fallen in love with lemon-water!

Looking back I realize this was actually quite a mountain for me. I had read from Matthew, "...if you have faith the size of a mustard seed, you will say to this mountain, 'move from here to there,' and it will move; and nothing will be impossible to you."

I believe I had been psychologically trained to order soft drinks whenever I was at a restaurant. Whether at a sit-down establishment or a fast-food outlet; when the server would ask, "May I take your drink order?" or "What drink would you like?" I somehow felt compelled to order a soda and ordering water felt strange; well not anymore!

The sensibility of ordering water has become crystal clear! It's good for me, it's refreshing and it's free! Why would I **not** order water?

I recently visited a friend and noticed that they had cases of soft drinks piled up on the floor from a recent food shopping trip. What was once normal for me now seemed strange. You see, when you get a revelation of something that helps you move towards your diet goals; it will make perfect sense to you but may seem very strange to others. I was not able to ask my friend why they had just bought so much unhealthy soft drinks! That would have been rude and very likely would have offended them. Not only that, but it also would have been hypocritical of me to criticize since I recently was doing the very same thing!

Sometimes when Jesus would heal someone, he would say to them: "...don't tell anybody..." You may want to keep you own specific diet solutions secret and instead just share the general concept so as not to upset anyone!

People often say that politics and religion are topics that are often too sensitive to discuss. Well you can add dieting to that list! Unless you are very close to someone, it is hard to bring up the topic of dieting in conversation. That's another reason why I wrote the Revelation Diet. Now I can simply and casually tell friends, "The ideas in this little book helped me a lot. Maybe you will like it too." This way, I don't have to ask questions. And when they ask me how I lost so much weight I can simply send them a copy.

Prayer for Chapter 3

"Dear God, thank you for the unique plans you have for me that will allow me to lose weight effectively and permanently. Help me to discover the best plans and follow them naturally as a part of my life." Amen.

Chapter 4 - Work It!

So now I had incorporated two simple principles; first I only ate wheat based products (bead or pasta) once per day and second, I started drinking water instead of juice or carbonated soft drinks. It wasn't long before I discovered a third. I read from Thessalonians "...if any would not work, neither should he eat." Now I know this is basically an admonition directed towards idleness but I read it and applied it towards my health and eating habits.

I thought, if I'm not working, then I should not be eating; and by working I thought of working out or exercising physically! (...a stretch in interpretation I know, but hey I was searching for answers!)

Getting back to physical 'work', have you ever wondered why marathon runners are almost always so slim? Simply because running is a permanent part of their lifestyle! If you talk to someone that runs marathons, it will not take long before you realize that running is at the forefront of their priorities. They arrange their schedule, their job, basically their whole life around their running schedule. Running is not something they fit into their schedule. Running is their life and everything else is forced to fit in around their running!

Now of course I don't recommend you decide to become a marathon runner. In fact I suggest that you refrain from 'taking up' any new drastic physical activity simply because it may be a temporary change and we want to find changes that are permanent.

Instead, see if there is a simple physical activity that can become a part of your routine. If you have to pack a gym bag with workout clothes, drive 20 minutes to a gym facility, then spend 30 minutes on a treadmill; how likely is it that you will be able to make this a consistent part of your daily routine? What if you were able to find a way to walk to work? Maybe you currently take a bus to work and you are able to change the drop off point so you are forced to walk the last fifteen minutes to your office. This is much more effective on a daily basis than trying to make it to the gym 3 times per week. This is what worked for me; I was able to incorporate a change that literally 'forced' me to exercise daily to get to where I needed to go. It was no longer exercise for the sake of exercise; it was now a necessary part of my schedule! In fact I was able to cancel my membership at the local gym which was costing me a monthly membership fee and I was not being consistent at the gym anyway!

This was the third pillar of change that was the tipping point for my weight loss. Combined with my strategy from Chapter Seven, it was basically the straw that broke the back of the overweight camel! You see, if you make one change in your lifestyle, you may not notice any change. If you make two changes, again, maybe your body will adapt and you will see no change or even continue to gain weight. But each time you make a small permanent change, you are adding one more factor in your favor that will eventually overwhelm your weight loss barrier.

If you have any experience with dieting at all, you will already know and appreciate how amazingly effective and efficient your body is at keeping weight on; it is this incredibly efficient design of our bodies that allows us to utilize what we eat for energy efficiently and to store energy for emergency.

Healthy permanent changes don't shock the body into a total 'conserve fat' mode. That's what often happens with 'crash' or 'fad' diets. You experience a temporary change but the body quickly adapts and goes back to its previous weight setting like a thermostat keeps the temperature constant.

Instead, healthy permanent changes allow your body to melt away fat naturally and progressively resulting in a leaner, healthier you!

Prayer for Chapter 4

"Dear God, please show me what physical activities I can add to my daily life that will help me lose weight and feel better at the same." Amen

Chapter 5 - Make It Happen!

Change is not easy. It takes effort. It takes effort to even ask for help! When you stop trying, you are done.

When was the last time you sincerely asked God for help? You should be asking for help every morning when you wake up. Believe for small victories. Don't let a single day go by without a small victory. You will have setbacks. You may go crazy at breakfast; the day is not over yet. You may have the dessert at lunch when you know you should have skipped it; the day is not over yet. You may feel too full at dinner; that's right, the day is not over yet!

If you are in a pattern of repeated failures, it means you are not planning ahead of the stopping point of your meals. What I mean is that some people go into a trance when they are sitting at a meal and don't wake up until 'it's over'. They lapse into a robot like state while eating and then regain consciousness and immediately think, "Whoa, I really overdid it that time." Don't let this be you!

Visualize the end of your meal first; that point when you have finished a healthy portion and are relaxing with a glass of water for dessert.

You don't just walk into the kitchen with the intention of fixing yourself a snack because you're hungry. That's like walking into a minefield because you want to take a short cut! Think ahead and plan each meal as an opportunity for victory. Before you sit down to eat, you want to visualize that you have just finished a healthy small meal that your body can easily digest and you are enjoying a glass of water; make this a habit.

If there are any items on your exclusion list, make sure you are avoiding those items. Did you have toast for breakfast? Fine, you have had your daily bread so now you plan that sandwich for lunch. You place the filling on a plate without the bread and you have an image of what you are going to have for lunch. Visualize, visualize, visualize! This cannot be over-emphasized because of the dangerous power of your auto-pilot habits.

If you will plan your meal ahead of time then you don't have to count calories because you will naturally choose a healthy meal and a small portion. It you start eating without thinking, it's like flipping a switch on a lawnmower and walking away! Where you come back, you're gonna have a nasty surprise. Instead, when you mow a lawn, you plan out how you are going to cut the corners in such a way that you have a beautiful result! The same is true when you are eating, plan ahead for a beautiful result. From Proverbs 16: "Commit your works to God and your plans will be established."

Prayer for Chapter 5

"Dear God, show me the way to victory in my eating habits. Show me the strategy that will work for me." Amen.

Chapter 6 – My Initial Revelation Diet Ideas.

The Revelation Diet can be a part of your mindset and lifestyle. It means that you will be on the lookout for permanent changes that you can make to your eating habits and physical activities. In my case, my Revelation Diet consisted of three simple changes that resulted in significant and permanent weight loss and then I found the total knockout strategy that I will discuss in the next chapter. The first was to have bread based foods only once per day. (Breads, pasta or other starchy wheat based food). The second was to drink only water in place of soda, coffee or tea. The third was that, due to re-locating, I was able to walk to work instead of driving.

Once you escape from calorie counting and torturing yourself every day with what you should or shouldn't eat or how much time you should spend on the treadmill, you will have a renewed energy in your life. You will be able to sense when God is showing you a personal strategy that will work for you. It is very exciting to find something that you know works for your own specific circumstances. As you pray for your own unique solutions, here are some strategies that you can prayerfully consider adding as a permanent change to your diet or lifestyle.

1. Eating only one per meal per day that contains bread or pasta.
2. Replacing carbonated soft drinks with water.
3. Walking to and from work.
4. Removing Refined White Sugar From Your Diet.
5. Switching to eating only whole wheat and/or whole grain bread instead of white bread.
6. Going for a fifteen minute walk on every lunch break.
7. Replacing butter in your diet with margarine or a low fat substitute.
8. Removing anything with hydrogenated vegetable oil from your diet.
9. Taking a fifteen minute walk or longer every morning before breakfast.

10. Drinking a large glass of water before every meal.

11. Eating a small garden salad as lunch at least once per week.

12. Fasting one day per week.

13. Doing a set number of pushups every morning upon waking.

14. Removing anything in your diet that contains nitrates.

15. Doing an activity regularly that you've always enjoyed like swimming or badminton.

16. Removing anything in your diet that contains caffeine.

17. Eating celery sticks as a late night snack at least once per week.

18. Switching to lower fat milk. Whole milk to 2% or 2% to skim milk etc.

19. Doing a set number of sit-ups every evening.

20. Replacing ice cream in your diet with a low fat substitute (frozen yogurt etc.)

You can see that the first three items on this list are things that I discovered worked for me. You can easily find many more. Every time you find a principle that works for you, write it down and add it to your own personal revelation diet list. One or two items will likely not make much difference in your life, but as you add more items, you will start to see some amazing results. Have fun with it and don't stop searching! Remember the admonition: "ask and you will receive"...scholars tell us that a good interpretation of this verse is to ask and *keep on asking*. "Seek and you will find". Again, seek and *keep on seeking*!

I used to love whole milk. Then I switched to 2% partially skim milk and I am used to it. Don't try and switch from whole milk to skim milk overnight; you will likely say, "bleeech" I can't drink that! You don't want to do anything that is too much of a shock to your taste-buds or body. Small gradual changes are easier to become permanent changes and that is what the Revelation Diet is all about. Discover those small permanent changes that are enjoyable and healthy for you personally.

You may have an idea; maybe you can take the stairs instead of the elevator. But if taking the stairs is painful and something you dread each day, it is unlikely to remain as a permanent change. Your changes should be exciting and fun and challenging but never painful.

God will make a way when there seems to be no way! From Isaiah 42 "I will lead the blind by a way they do not know, in paths they do not know I will guide them. I will make darkness into light before them and rugged places into plains. These are the things I will do, and I will not leave them undone." Have you been blind to a weight loss victory? Change that starting now!

Prayer for Chapter 6

"Dear God, help me to find permanent changes I can make in my diet and lifestyle that are enjoyable and improve my health while lowering my weight." Amen.

Chapter 7 – The Revelation Diet Breakthrough!

So now I went to get to something really exciting! You see, when I first got my weight under control using a few simple lifestyles changes like those discussed above; I still had a nagging feeling that I might be missing something. My body still had a few stubborn tricks up its' sleeve. It's hard to explain but I had the nagging suspicion that my body was not co-operating with me but was simple playing possum until it saw an opportunity for 'revenge'. More often than not, this would be either a family gathering, a special visit to a restaurant or an unexpected occasion of 'free food' that made me feel compelled to eat more than normal. These types of events had the effect of reversing weeks and weeks of disciplined eating. Was I still missing something? I went back to prayer.

I asked God to please open my eyes in case I was missing something. I must confess that I am not sure what my motivation was – perhaps it was vanity, perhaps it was simply watching the natural aging process within my own body; whatever the motivation, I was often absolutely filled with self-hatred and self-disgust and I begged God in case I was missing something.

Shortly thereafter, God must have answered my prayer and gave me the following eating plan. Now before I blurt out what worked for me, I need to repeat that this obviously is not something that will work for everybody. I am not a doctor – I am not a nutritionist; I am simply a desperate individual that was at my wits end and was praying for something that would work for me. This plan is so simple that I am worried you may scoff and dismiss it offhand but please hear me out to explain the details and perhaps even promise me to try it yourself for three days before making a judgment about it one way or the other!

The Revelation Diet

Breakfast:

One (1) Apple Sliced and eaten slowly.

Green Tea.

Water.

Lunch:

Any vegetarian meal.

Water.

Dinner:

One (1) Orange separated into pieces and eaten slowly.

Water.

Details:

You can drink any amount of green tea during the day.

No coffee.

No alcohol.

(I allowed myself to drink alcohol one day per week in moderation.)

Minimal dairy, since lunch is an 'open' meal, you may sometimes be having small amounts of cheese or milk with your lunch meal. Lunch can be anything but you will have better digestion and more energy with a balanced vegetarian meal that includes protein sources like nuts, tofu or beans.

'Lunch' can be any time of day from 11:00 AM to 5:00 PM. Some people who detest eating breakfast may have their Apple at around 11:00 AM and then not get hungry until 3 or 4 PM in the afternoon. Try and keep at least 3 or 4 hours between 'breakfast' and 'lunch' and 'dinner'.

If you get too hungry in the evening you can have a second or third orange with water or green tea; however, the great thing about this plan is that it seems to be very effective in reducing appetite.

So there you have it – this is something that came to me in a dream and I believe it was an answer to prayer. I tried it for a day and noticed that I did not get hungry in the evening. I tried it for three days and weight melted off me. I know it is a bit extreme so of course I need to strongly express the usual disclaimer.

Please see a doctor or a trained nutritional expert before trying any type of diet recommendation. I can only tell you about my personal experience and make no claim as to how this diet plan may affect the reader either positively or negatively.

That being said, I would love to hear feedback from anyone that might like to try this program for themselves. You can email me directly at patrick@patrickdoucette.com.

I wish I could provide you all sorts of scientific details about why this may be effective as a temporary weight loss plan but I am simply not qualified to do so – but think about it for a moment – even if I was trained in nutrition, there would be people who would immediately argue against it. For every new diet that comes out, there are also immediate naysayers whose opinion is in direct opposition to what is being recommended! That's why I am presenting this as something that is exciting and working for me but since every person is unique, I am hoping that you will be inspired to find your own unique solution.

Maybe you try this exact plan and it also works for you – nothing would make me happier than to discover that this plan indeed works for many people! And why not? – If it worked for me, there surely must be others who will also experience positive results.

When I had the dream of the above diet plan I saw an apple and I was thinking that it started with the letter 'A'. I saw the orange and it started with the letter 'O'. I immediately thought Alpha and Omega, the beginning and the end. An apple to start the day and an orange to end the day. Was this just a coincidence? Does that sound silly or corny to you? For me personally, it was a confirmation in my heart that this was something special, this was a unique plan that I could try and then share with friends and loved ones. I saw immediate benefits. Not only did I lose weight quickly but I also had more energy and my digestion was improved dramatically.

Both apples and oranges have appetite suppressing effects; perhaps they have appetite suppressing effects that have not even been discovered yet!

Experiment with the Revelation Diet – the lunch meal is open so perhaps at first, you will need to have a large meal with lots of protein; find what will allow you to get through the day feeling energized. Some days I have had one of those pre-washed Ceasar Salad kits as my lunch meal. Other days I have an order of vegetarian Pad Thai noodles. Still other days I have had a large vegetable stir-fry. I have come to cherish and savor the mid-day meal since obviously the other two 'meals' are pretty meager on this plan!

Again, I would suggest that you avoid dismissing this plan outright until you try it. An orange with a glass of water and then followed with a hot cup of green tea had a near miraculous effect of eliminating my late night food cravings. Prior to trying this diet, I would sometimes have a ravenous appetite in the evening – the Revelation Diet changed all that.

Maybe you can tweak it to your own taste. Maybe you can substitute a different type of tea that you prefer. Maybe you will try it and also get impressive results, fantastic! – that would also be great to hear!

Please try it for three days, tell me your results. Maybe you will be brave and try it for a week — maybe you will only need to follow the Revelation Diet Plan when you want to shed a quick few pounds without feeling overly hungry and while maintaining your energy level — I leave it to the reader as to how you want to best implement this simple Alpha and Omega strategy. Just remember beginning and end. You start the day with an apple and you end the day with an orange. What could be simpler? Sometimes, simple works!

Chapter 8 - Why This Will Work!

Early on in my process of discovering what works, I had read from Matthew, "...man (or woman) shall not live on bread alone, but by every word that proceeds forth from God." This is the essence of The Revelation Diet! It's not about the bread; **it's not about the food!** It's about a **word** of revelation that works for you! God promises to guide us as mentioned in Psalm 73 " ... with your counsel you will guide me..." and also in Isaiah 58 "...(God) will continually guide you, and satisfy your desire... and give strength to your bones..." Now that's what I call a powerful and encouraging revelation!

Most diet plans consist of a set of detailed guidelines or complicated instructions for you to follow. The reason why the Revelation Diet is different from every other diet is because even though it has a simple basic plan; the underlying theme is that you can and should also discover your very own principles to follow that are unique to you!

When you discover something for yourself, it is like receiving a personal gift of guidance from God. How much more will you cherish such a divine direction! Maybe there is a mountain in your life when it comes to a particular food. Maybe it's butter or ice cream; it doesn't matter; but for you it feels like a mountain that you just can't give up. The fact of the matter is that with God's help you can move that mountain! Maybe you will discover a substitute. Maybe just switching to a low fat alternative for ice cream is a permanent change you can implement in your life. You may discover a low fat version that is just as delicious; such a discovery alone can feel like a miracle!

When you discover a personal strategy that works for you, you may want to keep it a secret or you may want to share it with your close friends. I would suggest writing it down and save the details in a journal so you can build a list of ideas that help you on your journey.

You may still be telling yourself, "I can't change." But the fact that you are reading this book proves that the desire for change is already within you. Consider this text from 2 Corinthians 1: "...the things that I purpose, do I purpose according to the flesh, that with me there should be yes yes, and no no? For all the promises of God... are yes,... unto the glory of God ... Now he which establishes ...()...you , and has anointed (you), is God..."

The things that you purpose to do are possible with God's help! You already know that is true, with God all things are possible. And yet when it comes to our weight, how quickly we concede that we have no strength or that we cannot change...what nonsense! We have fooled ourselves into believing a lie. The truth is that you **can** effect change, permanent radical and life altering change is possible for everyone!

Prayer for Chapter 8

"Dear God, help me to believe that change is possible for me! Show me some strategies that will work for me." Amen.

Chapter 9 - Why You Can't Fail!

There is no failure with the Revelation Diet. Whether you follow the Revelation Diet plan for one day or many days in a row, you are simply on a constant path towards victory. Even if there are setbacks, every day is a new chance to discover a new solution that works for you.

You may want to start a Revelation Diet friendship group. You can meet together and share ideas of what is working for each individual. Everyone will have something unique that they will be able to share to encourage others. There is a certain comfort and strengthening that occurs when people share a difficult experience together.

You already know losing weight can often be a difficult experience. It would be nice if it wasn't. Sometimes you can find strategies that are painless and make a big difference. For example, I was amazed at how much more energy I had simply by not drinking sugared juice or soda anymore! But you also have to face the fact that there is a direct correlation between weight and food consumption; and because of this you may be facing the prospect of voluntarily being hungry on a consistent basis. This is something that goes contrary to our nature. We want to be satiated; we want to feel full because it gives us a sense of comfort and security. We were made this way and we can be thankful for it or we would have never survived past the baby bottle!

But choosing to be hungry can also be a victory. It is certainly not easy; in fact, I believe it takes a certain amount of mental re-programming to achieve this. I am guessing that if you watch television for more than one hour per day, it is probably not possible to enjoy being hungry. Why? Simply due to the amount of money and resources invested by food companies into programming you to eat! This is really a North American phenomenon. I spent a month living in South Korea and their television and media programming is much different. In South Korea the investment by advertisers is made in the area of beauty products such as skin care products and dental and cosmetic surgery. It was no surprise that my weight plummeted while I was there with no noticeable effort!

The principle of avoiding television could be a Revelation Diet principle that makes a huge impact on your weight loss program! Consider carefully what you are watching!

Sometimes you may want to eat something because it is leftover and you want to make sure "it doesn't go bad". This is really a nasty trap. You look in the refrigerator and you see food and so you say to yourself, "I better eat this up or it will go bad and I will have to throw it out." It is a commendable desire to not waste food when there are people in the world that are starving. You must get over this feeling of guilt of wanting to clean up scraps like a vacuum cleaner. Have you ever watched someone that is slim eat a hamburger? Watch closely, often they will take a few bites and leave half in the garbage. Why is that? I believe part of the reason is that they are programmed to detest the feeling of being full. They may have been born that way or maybe it's from habit. It doesn't matter why but it's something you can learn from them. You have to come to terms with the idea of wasting food as a trade-off in relation to your own health. Think of losing weight as a battle and you need a 'take-no-prisoners' attitude to be able to win. Burn the bridges and throw out the leftovers!

Have you ever been to an 'all you can eat' restaurant? You will invariably see overweight individuals consuming many plates of food. Don't go to an all you can eat buffet unless you have already achieved powerful self-discipline. Sometimes you can gain insights just by watching how slim people eat and copying what they do or by watching fat people eat and avoiding what they do. This may be harsh but it is reality. There are people that have already achieved what you are trying to accomplish; follow what they do. Don't listen to the infomercials that show testimonials of people holding up their old clothes. "I lost 200 pounds using the magic ab-dissolver exercise machine" or "I lost 150 pounds following these magic exercise videos." No, instead look around you; see the real people in your real neighborhood. See what the people in your immediate family are doing. What is working for them, what is not working?

Prayer for Chapter 9

"Dear God, help me to appreciate the feeling of being hungry since I know it is an indicator that I am achieving my dreams and goals! Grant me victory to lose weight." Amen.

Chapter 10 - Write It Down – Say It!

The Revelation Diet is essentially the path of discovery for what works for you as an individual so it is extremely valuable for you to track your own progress and achievements. Psalm 105 talks about how Joseph suffered in prison "until the time of his **word** came" then he was delivered and rose to great success. What is your word that is awaiting fulfillment? Have you written down your goals?

Someone once said that goals that are not written down are just fantasies or daydreams. Write out your goals. Try to practice writing out what you are planning to eat for your next meal. If you regularly sit down to eat and then wake up 40 minutes later and try and take stock of everything you have just eaten; you need to change! You want to be directing yourself and not just reacting.

Consider the verse from 1 Corinthians, "I control my body and bring it into subjection". That a reminder that you need to be the one in control of your body, not your body controlling you!

Not only are your written words powerful but also your spoken words. Watch closely to things that overweight people say. "I just love___(fill in the blank with any food)". They often say they love steak or they love a particular flavor of ice cream. **Never** say that you love food. I know a dear neighbor who once said to me; "I love it when my wife makes peach crumble, it's just to die for!" Guess what? Ironically this poor soul is dying from obesity related illnesses and he is oblivious to his own language of failure. He has complications from diabetes and will likely have a short life expectancy unless he makes radical changes in his eating habits. I'm ashamed to say I didn't have the heart nor the faith to try and suggest that he change the way he talks about food. It would probably be awkward, upset him and maybe I would have lost a friend.

Maybe you have a friend or a loved one like that too. Maybe they will read this and recognize themselves;

it could be a wake-up call that can save a life or at the very least radically improve it! Don't let it be you! Consider what Solomon said in Proverbs 18: "A man's belly shall be satisfied with the fruit of his mouth; and with the increase of his lips shall he be filled."

What comes out of our mouths is vitally important! Speak words of victory about your diet, speak words of victory about your strength to change and you will reap the rewards. Remember the parable from Luke 19, "...by your own words I will judge you..." This is a scary thought! We sow with our words and we reap our circumstances.

You may very well say, "But, I've heard it all before. I've read it all before. " Well, you may have heard it all before but have you said it all before? Have you prayed it all before? The road to weight loss victory can be a lonely road but you are not alone. God wants to help you. His plans are to help you succeed. From Jeremiah, "God says: For I know the thoughts that I think toward you, thoughts of peace, and not of evil, to give you an expected end. Then you will call upon me, and you shall pray unto me, and I will hearken unto you." Wow! Now that's what you can call a promise of victory! You may have heard that verse a dozen times before but have you let it sink in lately? God is saying He wants to listen to your prayers; He wants to restore your health and vitality!

Pray with passion like the words from 2 Chronicles: "(Dear God), have respect therefore to the prayer of your servant, and to my supplication ...my God, to hearken unto the cry and the prayer which your servant prays before you," grant me victory in my diet, show me and lead me along the way to healthy weight loss.

When you seek Gods help with genuine sincerity, how can you possibly fail? The only way you can fail is if you give up, so...don't give up! Ask God to help you and He will!

There are so many ways to lose weight. Medically assisted diet regimens, surgical procedures, powerful drugs, proven diet strategies and techniques. You may already have a plan in place that you know works but are unable to stick to it. This is exactly when you need a revelation from a God; a divine intervention that breaks through the chain that has been holding you back from success. The result is worth the effort! You have your health and energy to gain! You have an extended lifespan to share with your family and loved ones. You have increased self-esteem and confidence. And of course we never mentioned your looks! Yes, when you lose weight you will look better but that is way down on the list of benefits; when you look closely at the results of a healthy diet you will see more important benefits than your looks!

Now we all know it's important to accept and love yourself no matter what size or shape you are; that's a given. The Revelation Diet is for those that have that deep down nagging feeling that they 'should' be eating better or eating less than they are now. They just haven't had the right motivation to take action or they just never prayed seriously about it. Will you start your own Revelation Diet today? Will you earnestly pray and ask God to show you what you can do that will work for you? I encourage you to start today; start today and never stop!

You will gradually draw closer and closer to your goals every day until you reach a point of powerful confidence and victory. You can do it!

Prayer for Chapter 10

"Dear God, help me to write down diet goals that can and will be achieved and help me to speak only words of victory." Amen.

Afterword

The goal of this book has been to help, encourage and inspire, but if the encouragement stops with you, how will others benefit? Because this book is published without any marketing or advertising budget; there's one small thing I need to ask. Can you take a moment or two and share this Revelation Diet message so others can benefit? My vision is to share this short gentle message with as many people as possible. I know in the natural this is a difficult task but I also know that with God all things are possible!

All I ask is that you consider one of the following action items to help spread the hope and encouragement.

1   Share a message about The Revelation Diet on your Facebook.

2   Tweet a message about the Revelation Diet to your twitter followers.

3   Send a free copy of The Revelation Diet to a friend or loved one.

4   Post a link to The Revelation Diet on your blog or web page.

I know there are many people out there that are struggling with their weight. They are taking two steps forward and three steps back. Maybe all they need is a slight boost in the right direction. You can provide that boost! Consider sending a gift copy of this book to someone you know; it would a delightful and encouraging surprise! For about the cost of a cup of coffee you can brighten someone's day and perhaps be the turning point in them achieving a new resolve in the battle against uncontrolled eating habits! Maybe you know someone that has given up the hope of ever being at a healthy weight. Perhaps they will find just one single idea from this short book that will be the trigger, the spark that starts a flame of victory! What a blessing that would be for you and for them – that is my hope!

Thank you for your consideration. It has been an honor to be able to share this message with you.

~ Patrick Doucette